Reverse Diabetes

A Step by Step Guide to Reverse Diabetes and Free Yourself from Stress, Anxiety, and Pain

Nancy Perez

Introduction

I want to thank you and congratulate you for purchasing the book, *"Reverse Diabetes: A Step by Step Guide to Reverse Diabetes and Free Yourself from Stress, Anxiety, and Pain"*.

Diabetes is a condition that can really drag anyone down - from having extra abdominal fat, experience urinary changes, elevated blood sugar, injuries that take a long time to heal, and so much more. This is why you have to make sure that you don't let diabetes take over your life —and that you work to reverse its effects.

Well, if you're reading, this then you have come to the right place.

This book contains proven steps and strategies on how to reverse the effects of diabetes—from how you should tweak your diet, why burst exercises work, and so much more—you'll find them all right here. With them, you'll not only get rid of diabetes, you can say goodbye to stress, and pain for good, too!

Read this book now and get yourself in the path of good health once more.

Thanks again for downloading this book, I hope you enjoy it!

Table of Contents

What is Diabetes?

Diabetes is a serious, chronic disease where your body is unable to process the glucose from your blood into the cells where they can use it for energy. As a result the glucose level in the blood is increased and the cells are not getting the glucose they need.

A lot of Americans have this disease (around 17 million) and almost one-third of them don't even know that they have it.

The food that we eat is divided into macro and micro nutrients. The macro nutrients are carbohydrates, proteins and fats while the micro nutrients include vitamins and minerals. Each of these play an important role in the functioning of the human body. The carbohydrates are used as an energy source, the fats are used for the health of the brain and organs while the proteins are used for muscle synthesis.

The carbohydrates are broken down into what we call glucose. This glucose is then circulated in the blood stream to provide energy to the cells of the body or to be stored for later use.

In order to use the glucose in such a way, the body makes use of insulin that is created in the pancreas. The cells in the pancreas increase or decrease insulin production based on the glucose levels in your blood stream. So when the glucose levels in the blood are high, they need to release more insulin to keep it in check. And this causes the other cells in the body to start consuming the glucose as energy. As a result the glucose levels in the blood will start returning to normal levels which in turn will reduce the amount of insulin that is being produced.

The problem of diabetes is that it causes a havoc with this process and therefore decreases the body's ability to regulate insulin in a balanced way.

The amount of harm diabetes causes to the body depends on the type of diabetes one is suffering from.

Diabetes needs to be treated with care as it can be a life-threatening disease among some of the other impacts it can have on your body such as blindness, gangrene, excessive urination, hunger and thirst.

Types Of Diabetes

There are three different kinds of diabetes known as Type 1, Type 2 and gestational diabetes.

Type 1 Diabetes

This type of diabetes cn occur at any age and is also known as juvenile diabetes. It generally occurs before the age of 20 and is supposedly rare affecting around five percent of people.

The main cause of this type of diabetes is that the body is unable to manufacture insulin because it lacks the beta cells that are required for this purpose.

This type of diabetes can happen due to genetics or even due to a viral attack where the beta cells are being destroyed. Some research scientists also believe that it might be the body's immune system itself attacking and destroying the beta cells.

The major problem with this type of diabetes is that since the beta cells are destroyed they cannot be recreated and so it's a lifetime disease. So patients with type 1 diabetes will require regular insulin injections. This type of diabetes cannot be prevented.

Type 1 diabetes has symptoms like tiredness, weight loss, excessive urination, itchiness and thirst.

Complications that may arise due to type 1 diabetes may include ketoacidosis and hypoglycemia. It can also cause kidney problems, stroke and heart ailments.

Type 2 Diabetes

This type of diabetes affects overweight people especially when they are old. Having a lazy or sedentary lifestyle is one of the contributing factors for such a type of diabetes. This lifestyle is causing problems not just in old but even among young people and children.

Almost 90% of diabetics suffer from the type 2 diabetes. It is also possible that some cases of this type of diabetes is hereditary.

In this type of diabetes, the body is able to generate the normal amounts of insulin but is unable to utilize the insulin to regulate the blood sugar levels. This condition is also known as insulin resistance. As a result of high blood sugar levels, the cells of the body get damaged.

Some of the symptoms of type 2 diabetes includes excessive thirst, frequent urination, vomiting, vision problems, weight loss, slow healing of wounds, excessive hunger and tiredness.

The onset of type 2 diabetes is slower compared to the type 1 diabetes and some people may have the disease but not even show the symptoms.

The treatment for type 2 diabetes involves an

improvement in the lifestyle and dietary habits as well as addition of exercise to the daily life. Medication may be required in situations where symptoms and the disease are causing health problems. In the worse cases, insulin injections are also required.

Gestational Diabetes

Gestational diabetes is a type of diabetes that can occur during pregnancy. This can be caused by hormone fluctuations during the second or third trimester of pregnancy.

It can affect around 2-10% of pregnancies and may be common in women whose family has a history of diabetes. This type of diabetes is temporary and goes away after child birth if the lifestyle and diet is taken care of correctly.

Some common symptoms include vomiting and tiredness.

It may cause complications like the babies having a high weight and requiring Cesarean section.

Factors That Influence Diabetes

Smoking

The risk of diabetes is increased in smokers due to the inflammation it causes in the body. Smoking also increases the level of glucose in the blood and hence can worsen the insulin resistance.

Obesity

This is the number one risk factor for causing diabetes. Most people diagnosed with type 2 diabetes are obese. These people are also physically inactive that compounds this problem further.

Diet

Saturated fats are one of the factors that can influence risk of diabetes. Having a diet low in fiber can also contribute to this risk. Beverages and fruit juices high in sugar also influence the risk of diabetes.

Change Your Diet

More than anything, you have to start making necessary changes to your diet. If you are a diabetic, you have to remember that it's your responsibility to make sure you're following a diet that's good for you, and that would not make your condition worse.

What Needs to Be Removed

You can start by removing certain food items from your diet—and of course, your grocery list. If you have the following items stored in your cupboards or the fridge, make sure that you remove them, too.

The following items are:

1. **Grains.** It would be best to go on a gluten-free diet. This is because grains contain a huge amount of carbohydrates, and carbohydrates may also contain a lot of sugar in them. More so, carbohydrates are easily turned into sugar once the body absorbs it. For the first 90 days after being diagnosed with diabetes, or at least, for your own "healing program", it would be best to say goodbye to grains.

2. **Refined Sugar.** Refined sugar is definitely not good for you because it brings forth a kind of sugar surge that could really elevate the amount of glucose in your bloodstream. Therefore, if you

want to sweeten whatever it is that you're eating, it would be best to go for Stevia instead, because maple syrup and honey spike up glucose levels, too.

3. **Canola, Soy, GMO Corn.** These are mostly found in packaged foods. They aren't good because they elevate blood sugar levels, and have also been linked to liver and kidney diseases.

4. **Alcohol.** Alcohol may worsen diabetes, and may also heighten the risk of liver cirrhosis and toxicity of the liver.

5. **Conventional Cow's Milk.** Cow's milk could prevent the body's immune responses from working properly, just like gluten does. If you're going to drink milk, take note that it might be better to go for sheep or goat's milk, instead.

Eat More of the Following

If you're going to remove certain food items from your diet, you also have to eat more of certain foods. For this, you have the following;

1. **Low-Glycemic Foods.** These are foods that won't spike up your blood sugar levels. Examples include *low pastured dairy, wild salmon, wild trout, eggs, organic meat, coconut, avocados, seeds, nuts, and vegetables.*

2. **Wild-Caught Fish**. Speaking of wild fish, what you can keep in mind about them is that they could reduce the levels of inflammation by a mile. It also prevents the body from experiencing the negative effects of glucose.

3. **MCFAs.** These are foods with medium chain fatty acids that balance your blood sugar levels so you won't suffer too much from diabetes. These are mostly found in *red palm oil and coconut oil*, as well.

4. **Chromium-Rich Foods.** These improve the body's tolerance for glucose, and also naturally balance the glucose-levels. Examples include *broccoli, grass-fed beef, green beans, and raw cheese.*

5. **Fiber-Rich Foods.** Fiber-rich foods help slow the body's absorption of glucose. 30 grams of fiber each day is already good. Examples include *seeds, nuts, berries, avocados, and vegetables.*

Good Fats

Good Fats are also a big part of the diabetic diet—so make sure that you eat the following:

1. **Flaxseed.** Flaxseed is considered as a super food because it is full of fiber, which, as you may know by now is important in an anti-Diabetic diet. Choose golden or yellow ones as they are healthier

than the others but otherwise, they're all good, too.

2. **Avocados.** Avocados are popular for being good sources of healthy fat. They do not only prevent and lower the risk of type II diabetes, they are good for the heart, too—which isn't something you can say for most types of fatty foods.

3. **Canola Oil.** Canola Oil lowers the level of bad cholesterol, or LDL in your bloodstream so you won't be at risk of the bad effects of diabetes or heart diseases and that's why it is considered as one of the best cooking oils around.

4. **Nuts.** Nuts are rich in protein and calcium, two of the most important minerals that you need. They also contain omega-3 fatty acids, L-arginine, and have vitamin E that prevents plaque accumulation so your blood can easily flow around your body, and prevent coronary heart diseases.

5. **Olive Oil.** Olive oil not only adds great flavor to your dishes, it's also something that is considered as one of the world's healthiest cooking oils because it is high in fiber and low in fat—and that's exactly the reason why it's used for most diet plans and dishes that you see.

6. **Tuna.** Tuna is full of omega-3 acids that are good for the heart and are also full of mono and poly-saturated fats that help control your glycemic

index. 2 to 3 servings each week will already do you a lot of good.

7. **Salmon.** And, just like tuna, salmon is also full of omega-3 acids, as well as omega-6 acids that your body certainly needs. More so, it is considered as one of the leanest kinds of fish out there, which makes it perfect for an anti-diabetic diet.

Sample Meal Plan

To easily understand the kind of diet that you should follow, try to follow this meal plan below:

Day 1

Breakfast: coconut smoothie

Lunch: chicken and spinach salad with olive oil and apple cider vinegar

Snacks: ¼ cup raw almonds

Dinner: grass-fed beef burger

Day 2

Breakfast: vegetable omelet with goat cheese

Lunch: chicken vegetable soup (made with real broth)

Snacks: 2 oz raw cheese

Dinner: grilled wild salmon with garlic

Day 3

Breakfast: peach probiotic shake

Lunch: turkey burger with small salad

Snacks: raw vegetables with guacamole

Dinner: chicken vegetable stir-fry

Try Burst Training

Of course, it's not just all about dieting. You have to train your body to be stronger, too. For that, you can make use of burst training exercises.

The great thing about burst training is that it helps you burn up to 3x more body fat than other exercises that you probably have been doing. It's also great because you have the choice to do the exercises at home.

Aside from that, burst training also provides you with more lean muscle and also speeds up your metabolic rate—you just have to do it 20 to 30 minutes a day and you're good.

Here are some exercises that you could try:

1. **High Jumps:** Stand in place, reach as far as you can above your head and jump as high as you can —you don't have to measure it, just jump as high as you can—and do it for at least 30 to 60 seconds.

2. **Run in place:** Run in place as fast as you can and make sure your knees are also as high as possible for this to make sense.

3. **Swim:** If you have a swimming pool at home, you can try burst or speed swimming. If not, maybe you can ask a friend to burst-swim with you at the community pool or at a swimming center, if

possible.

4. **Bike:** Try cycling indoors by spin-cycling, or take your bike outdoors and bike as fast as you can. Make sure you're in a safe area where motorists don't pass by, though, so you can be sure that you'll be safe.

5. **Jump Rope:** Have some fun and start playing jump rope again.

6. **Squat Pulses:** Get in a position where your feet are at least a shoulder-distance apart. Squat as low as you can and then move up and down. Don't allow your knees to move past your toes.

7. **Jumping Jacks:** Finally, you can try good old jumping jacks! Try to do this as much as you can for at least 30 seconds to see how many you can do.

With the help of these exercises, you'll get a good rush of adrenaline, improve your heart rate by a whopping 90 to 100%, and lessen the effects of diabetes for good.

Say Goodbye to Plastic

Next, you have to make necessary lifestyle changes, one of which is finally saying goodbye to the use of plastic. The reason for this is that plastic contains common chemicals, known as *phthalates* that double the risk of type II diabetes. These are mostly found in vinyl products, perfumes, toys, packaging, personal care products, cosmetics, clothing, and other building materials.

Of course, it's not expected that you'd say goodbye to all those things altogether—especially because you do need them in your life. However, it would be good if you can make use of alternatives—and be conscious in not patronizing the use of plastic. For this, you can keep the following in mind:

Ventilate Your Home

Ventilating your home is good because it lessens the effect of phthalate levels that are prevalent indoors. Open more windows, and let natural air in. It would be good if you can plant outside so fresh air would really be around the house. Try making use of structural ventilation for upward air flow, or roof ventilation so air wouldn't be too hot. Try to diffuse some lavender or vanilla-scented oils around the house, too.

Avoid Products with the #3 symbol

This means that the product—or its plastic packaging—is made from PVC, which is also known as plastic that contains additives that can be harmful for your body.

Buy Phthalate-Free Products

These also include fragrance-free ones. There are so many beauty products that work great even without phthalate—so make sure that you keep them in mind! Examples include *Juice Beauty, Iredale Mineral Cosmetics, Herbalix Restoratives, Exfoliating Minerals, Colby Organic, and Coastal Classic Creations*, among others.

Try Plastic Alternatives

Possibly the best thing you can do is really make the necessary change of using plastic alternatives. Here are some examples:

1. **Glass.** Glass is a great container. Not only is it decorative, it also does not contain any harmful elements that can make its way through your food or your body—unless it's crushed, of course. Glass also doesn't melt in the microwave the way plastic does.

2. **Reusable Shopping Bags.** Reusable shopping bags are much more convenient to use because of the fact that well, you can use them over and over again. Using plastic bags is not only bad for your body, it's not good for the environment, as well.

There are over 1 billion plastic bags that are being used in the United States alone—and just less than 1% is being recycled! Just think of what that's doing to the environment—and how it could affect you. When the environment is filled with plastic, there are more chances that your body would be affected by what phthalates could do—and that's never a good thing.

On the other hand, reusable shopping bags could also be quite fashionable. They come in a variety of styles—nylon, canvas, cotton, hemp, and sometimes, even leather! This way, you won't feel like you're compromising your style as you're trying to protect yourself.

3. **Milk Protein.** Milk protein could be turned into clothes and shoes—and some fashion designers are already doing so these days. What's great about these products is that they contain casein—a biodegradable material that's been proven to be good for the body and the environment, as well. It has also been around since the 1800s, and is proven to be less susceptible to cracking. It somehow feels like polyester without being too stingy.

4. **Liquid Wood.** Liquid wood is currently being processed these days as a byproduct of water and paper mills. It has a non-toxic and strong composition that can withstand heat—the way

certain plastic materials don't. The best part is that they are biodegradable—so you know you'd get to help your body and the environment, as well. Liquid wood is usually used for Hi-Fi speaker boxes, golf tees, and certain toys.

By saying goodbye to plastic, you're able to live a better, healthier reality.

Try Yoga and Breathing Exercises

Yoga is not just for exercise or meditation experts. Yoga helps reduce the risk of diabetes because it helps the abdomen relax. Furthermore, it also naturally alternates the release of pancreatic juices, and abdominal contractions that then increase oxygen and blood supply in the body.

When there's fresh blood flow in your body, your liver gets to produce more insulin, which of course, is used to prevent and treat diabetes. Breathing exercises related to yoga also stimulate the health of the pancreas.

Diabetes also prevents the effects of hypoglycemia, or the surge in glucose levels that is one of the main causes of diabetes. It lessens triglyceride levels, as well.

Poses to Try

Here are the best yoga poses against diabetes:

1. **Bridges**. Lie on the floor and bend your knees over the heels. Exhale with your arms at your sides, then lift your hips and make sure that they are parallel to the floor. Hold this position for at least a minute.

2. **Dog Gone Yoga.** Go on all fours with your hands

under your shoulders, and with your knees under your hips; then walk forward with your knees curled under and hold 3 full breaths.

3. **Mountain Yoga.** Do this by standing with your shoulders relaxed and your feet together, then raise your hands upwards, take a deep breath, and reach towards the sky.

4. **Perfect Pigeon.** In a push-up position, let your palms align with your shoulders then place your left knee on the floor, perpendicular to your shoulder. Bring your right leg down and lower your forearms and make sure that your chest is just right in front of you. Now, bring your chest towards the floor and pull your navel in, while curling your toes. Bend your knees for around 5 reps toward the floor and repeat on the other side of your body.

5. **The Child.** Sit comfortably then roll your body forward, alongside your forehead. Then, as low as you can, lower your chest by extending your arms forward. Breathe and hold this position for 5 to 10 breaths.

6. **The Crow.** Do the "dog" position and walk directly northwards until your arms are able to touch your knees. Then, lift your heels off the floor and bend your elbows. Rest your knees against your upper arms for around 5 to 10 breaths with your legs and abs against your arms.

7. **The Snake.** On the floor, lay face-down and tighten your pelvis on the floor. Squeeze your glutes and tuck your hips, then make sure that your shoulders are pointing away from your ears. Push your index fingers and thumbs down and inhale. Repeat as much as you can because this will help you relax.

8. **Tree Yoga.** With your arms at your sides, stand up and make sure to shift your weight to the left leg. Bring your hands in the position of a prayer in front of you and inhale for around 30 seconds. Repeat on the left side.

9. **True Triangle.** Extend your arms to both sides and bend your right leg. With your feet at a 90 degree angle and with your toes apart, touch the floor with your right hand and extend your fingertips towards the ceiling. Hold this stance for at least 5 seconds and gaze towards the ceiling, then repeat on the opposite side of your body.

10. **Twist and Sit.** Extend your legs while sitting on the floor, then cross your right leg over the left and place your left elbow next to the right knee. Twist your body for as far as you can and stay in that position for a minute.

11. **Warrior Type.** With your legs 3 to 4 feet apart, do a 90 degree angle to the right with your left foot in, and then relax your shoulders after bringing them down to your hips. Bend your knees

and gaze to the right, then repeat with your left side.

12. **Lingering Breath**. Sit down on the floor in a cross-legged position. Inhale slowly and exhale on the count of 5. Inhale for another 5 counts, and exhale the same way. Continue for at least 3 sets.

Breathing Exercises

And of course, here are the breathing exercises that you can try to accompany your yogic poses:

Channeling GOD

1. Use your thumb to touch each of your fingers, and imagine the planets coming together for your benefit.

2. Stretch your arms up to 60 degrees upwards. Open your fingers and spread them apart widely. Make sure they are hard, and then cross your arms in alternating motion. You'd feel some pressure on your spine now.

3. Say GOD 3 times, thinking that he Generates, Organizes, Delivers, as well as Destroys. Open yourself up to those thoughts and bask in them.

4. Relax. Allow yourself to forget what needs to be forgotten, and to just focus on the now. Whisper strongly with the thought that you want all

diseases to be burned.

5. Put your hands together, shoulder-width apart, with the left hand under and the right one over. Make long and deep breaths and don't let your hands fall down.

6. Keep your spine straight and sit down for a minute, and just focus on your breathing. Take 20 seconds to inhale, 20 to exhale, and so on.

7. Breathe consciously until you notice that you feel so much better—even with the pressure on.

Thumb and Breathing

1. Use your thumb and index finger to pinch your eyebrows.

2. Massage your temples.

3. Pull your ears for at least 10 to 15 seconds. The reason for doing this is simple: yogis believe that doing so is also a sign that says that no other person will be.

4. Close your eyes, then open them wide. Use your fingers to pull them wide and do massage your chin and cheeks by using your first, middle, and ring fingers.

5. Move your ears clockwise and counter-clockwise.

6. For around 8 to 10 times, move your jaws.

7. Take a few deep breaths and move your head to the motion.

Easing the tension

1. Lie down on a bed or sit on a reclining chair and do the following:

2. Focus on one part of your body, such as the left leg or the left arm.

3. For at least 5 seconds, take a deep breath and squeeze the muscles on that area. Don't worry if you feel uncomfortable—you're supposed to release some tension, anyway, but of course, make sure that the pain is bearable and that it doesn't feel like pain is shooting up from the inside. Listed below are some of the ways you can "squeeze" various parts of your body:

4. Raise shoulders towards your ears

5. Take a deep breath to tighten the chest

6. Shut your eyelids tightly

7. Stretch your jaw by opening your mouth wide

8. Raise eyebrows as high as possible

9. Pull toes towards you to tighten calf muscles

10. Curl toes downward

11. Squeeze thigh muscles

12. Draw forearms toward your shoulder

13. Clench fists

14. Inhale to tuck your stomach in

Getting Zen

1. First, just sit down and remain in the present moment. Don't even think about what you're going to do. Don't think about yesterday or tomorrow— just stay in the present moment. Once you do so, you'll be able to calm your mind and just be who you really are.

2. Then, you can focus all of your attention on the way your breath moves in and out of your nose. You can count from 1 to 100 with your mind and then move back again (100, 99, 98... etc.) When you get back to 1 you can count from 100 again and vice versa. This trick really calms the mind down and helps you stay in the present moment so you'd stop thinking about trivial things that just drive you down.

By trying these exercises, you not only protect yourself against diabetes, you also get to have a better, stronger body.

Read Nutritional Labels

Next, you have to keep in mind that it's also your responsibility to be mindful of Nutritional Labels. Yes, it might take a bit of your time and you may feel that maybe it's a bit complicated, but learning how to read nutritional labels is crucial to fighting diabetes.

Here's what you have to keep in mind:

Check for Fiber Amount

High-fiber foods work great in reversing the effects of diabetes, as mentioned earlier. Always check if the food product you have on hand has 3 or more grams of fiber contained in it. For this, you have to count carbohydrates by subtracting half the total amount of fiber from the carbohydrates to see if you'd get 3 grams or more. If you do, it means that your body will be able to keep itself from absorbing more carbohydrates than needed.

Total Carbohydrates vs. Sugar

Make sure that you compute for the amount of total carbohydrates. These include fiber, complex carbohydrates, and sugar, compared to just grams of sugar found in one product. By counting the right amount of carbohydrates, you would subject yourself to eating foods with natural or no sugar added, and you'd also be getting a good fill of carbohydrates—minus the effects of sugar.

What Sugar Really Means

Sugar could really make or break you, especially if you have diabetes because reading it could be tricky.

For example, when a label says that a product is "sugar-free", it usually means that it has less than 0.5 grams of sugar contained in it. In short, you don't necessarily have to choose the "sugar-free" product alone because there are times when its carbohydrate content may be larger than products with some sugar in them—so again, you have to count carbohydrates.

Sugar Alcohols also are not sugar-free because they have some calories and complex carbohydrates in them. Examples include *mannitol, xylitol, and sorbitol.*

Fat-Free Is not Carbohydrate-Free

Some products promote themselves as "fat-free", but actually, these would do nothing good for you because sometimes, they contain as many calories as carbohydrate-filled ones.

Besides, it's the sugar that you really have to keep track of—because there are food products with good fats that could protect you from diabetes, as mentioned in the first chapter.

Speaking of which, remember that it would always be

good to go for *polysaturated* or *monosaturated* fats—AKA the good fats—because *trans* and *saturated* fats only increase the risk of diabetes and heart disease.

Free-Foods

Free foods are those kinds of foods that have less than 5 grams of carbohydrates, and less than 20 calories per serving. You can have as much of these as you like. They are: *sugar-free gum, sugar-free flavored gelatin, and diet sodas.*

Calorie Goals and Serving Sizes

Lastly, you have to consider your daily calorie goals, as well as the serving sizes of the food you're trying to eat. Take note that serving sizes are based on a 2000-calorie diet, so 20% of anything is high, and 5% or less is low.

You also have to remember that nutritional values are based on serving size alone. When you double the serving size, you double the amount of calories, fats, or whatever it is that you'll be getting, as well.

The next time you shop for food, make sure that you keep the given tips in mind.

Get Some Shut-Eye

And of course, getting a good amount of sleep is important if you want to reverse the effects of diabetes and live a stress-free life.

However, it's not uncommon for people these days to get an insufficient amount of sleep because life is often busy and full of work. But, there are still certain guidelines that you can follow to help you get a good night's rest—and keep your health in check, as well.

For this, keep the following in mind:

Control Light Exposure

What most people fail to realize is that the amount of light in a room can really prevent them from going to sleep. To control light exposure, make sure that you follow these tips below:

1. **Let natural light get in the house during daytime.** This way, you'd get your fill of light especially when working at home.

2. **Only expose yourself to bright light early in the morning—if you can.** Try having breakfast or coffee outside, especially early in the morning when sunlight is still healthy for your skin.

3. **Use a light therapy box.** This stimulates sunlight

during the winter season.

4. **Don't watch TV at night.** At night, make it a point not to watch TV anymore. If you're getting bored, try to read a book instead. Light from the TV suppresses melatonin—the hormone that helps you get to sleep—and could even make you anxious—and that's not what you like to happen.

5. **Choose a good night reader.** If you're into reading eBooks, make sure that you choose a reader that won't give out too much bright light at night, such as *Nook Glowlight* or *Kindle Paperwhite*.

6. **Keep the lights down.** Or at least, dim the lights if you are afraid of the dark. Sleeping in a dark room still proves to be way more relaxing than sleeping in a room full of light. Dark puts your mind into "sleep mode".

Follow Your Natural Rhythm

This means that you have to make sense of your biological clock. If you sleep at the same time each day —even on weekends—then your body would have a good natural rhythm, and you'd be more in control of it. You also would reverse the effects of diabetes because your body won't easily get stressed out.

1. **Go to sleep at the same time each day and avoid sleeping in**. Try to choose a time when you

know you already feel tired. For example, you try to sleep by 9 but you know you still have way too much energy—so it just won't work. Choose a time you're more comfortable with, instead, such as 11PM—and sleep at that time. Avoid sleeping in because it'll just make you feel lazy—and would prevent you from exercising or doing yoga.

2. **Nap smartly.** 15 to 20 minutes is already good. Do not go overboard because it would ruin your natural rhythm.

3. **Do something stimulating after dinner**. This way, you could prevent after-dinner drowsiness and you'd get to sleep on your chosen time. Try calling a friend, reading a book, or preparing your clothes for the next day instead.

Improve Your Environment

Make sure your bedroom is somewhere that allows you to sleep. For this, you can follow these tips below:

1. **Comfortable sheets and pillows.** Try memory foam pillows, and blankets made of plush cotton or silk. Try cool colors so they would be soothing to the eyes—none of those overly-geometric designs, or pillows in hot pink or flame red.

2. **Keep the room cool.** If you can, adjust the thermostat to 18 C or 65 F—this is considered as the best temperature that allows people to sleep

without any hassle.

3. **Keep the noise down**. Just try to eliminate as much noise as you can. Try making use of a white noise machine, or meditative recordings to help you clear your head before you sleep. Speaking of which...

Clear Your Head

Sometimes, you really just have to help yourself. In order to sleep better, you have to clear the noise in your head.

1. **Visualize a serene place**. What's a place that keeps you relaxed? Try to visualize it. It could be a beach, or a hammock, or a grand bedroom with lights that are dimmed. Instead of counting sheep, visualize this place to help you become sleepy.

2. **Progressive relaxation**. Try progressive relaxation. This one has a lot to do with your muscles. Mostly, you should sit in a room with loose clothing and with good ventilation. Breathe deeply in and out and just relax before turning your attention to the right foot. Focus on how your right foot feels, and then tense the muscles on the said foot. Squeeze as tight as you can. Focus on how the tension feels like, and also how it goes away, and then bring your attention to the left foot. Relax for a moment, and breathe slowly and deeply.

Be Mindful of What You'd Eat and Drink

And of course, you have to be mindful of what's in your stomach before you sleep, which means that...

1. **Avoid drinking too much liquid before bed—especially alcohol**. Liquids could just make you pee so much, but of course, if you know you'd get dehydrated, do get a good amount of water in your system. However, you have to avoid alcohol because it would just interfere with your sleep cycle—and that's not what you want to happen.

2. **Don't eat big meals at night**. Try not to eat fatty food in the evening, or at least 2 to 3 hours before going to bed because it just might increase the risk of getting nightmares or suffering from acute pancreatitis. It would also do nothing good for your metabolism, and you need to increase metabolic rate if you want your diabetes to be healed.

3. **Don't drink caffeine**. Caffeine causes sleeping problems even 12 hours before sleeping time—so just imagine what it would do to your body a mere few minutes before going to bed! Cut back on the caffeine not just at night—but cut back on your overall intake.

Keep these tips in mind and you'll surely lessen the risk of diabetes.

BONUS

Superfoods And Recipes To Reverse Diabetes And Feel Healthy, Energetic And Happy

Introduction

Diabetes affects millions of people all around the world. It is an epidemic that spares no one. Even small children are being diagnosed with diabetes.

The problem is brought about by various reasons. Food is a huge factor in the development of type 2 diabetes.

The components of what you eat have direct effects on your blood sugar. Some foods cause blood sugar to rise almost immediately. Some foods help maintain stable blood sugar levels. Some foods cause hormones like insulin to get out of control. Some foods promote better hormonal regulation.

This book will teach what foods are best to reduce risk for diabetes. These superfoods can also help improve diabetic conditions. Find out what these foods are and how these can help you or the people around you.

You also get some bonus recipes to get you started on eating diabetes-friendly meals. These meals are savory, decadent, rich and flavorful. Diabetic diets do not mean bland, unappetizing foods. You can still enjoy wonderful food without damaging your tissues. Read on and be enlightened.

How Diet Can Be Used To Reverse Diabetes

There are a lot of superfoods that can help diabetics. These superfoods contain nutrients that help in various ways. Some of these can help improve or reduce insulin sensitivity. Some can help with better sugar control. Some can help in improving sugar metabolism. Some act on receptor cells for better insulin and blood sugar regulation.

These superfoods can easily be worked into the rest of the diabetic diet. These can be used as toppings to add texture to food. These can be added to give more depth of flavor or a new twist to everyday meals. There are so many ways to use more of these superfoods in the diabetic diet and get their benefits.

How Superfoods Help

Superfoods work in various ways to help improve the symptoms of diabetes. Some of the key actions include:

- Low glycemic index

  These foods are low GI, which means these do not cause large fluctuations in blood sugar levels.

- High in nutrients

  These superfoods supply the body with key

nutrients that are commonly lacking in the typical Western diet. The deficiencies contribute largely to poor regulatory mechanisms and cellular communication in the body. This in turn contributes to the development and worsening of diabetes. These superfoods provide a good amount of nutrients such as fiber, potassium, vitamins A, E and C, magnesium and calcium.

- Antioxidants

The antioxidants help to clear the system of free radicals and toxins that interfere with normal regulatory mechanisms. Antioxidants also protect the cells against oxidative damage. This type of damage also contributes to insulin resistance and diabetes.

Super-foods That Help To Reverse Diabetes

BEANS

Any type of bean is a superfood for diabetics. Your choices include black beans, navy, pinto or kidney beans. Beans are high in fiber and good source of potassium and magnesium. A half-cup serving of beans already gives 1/3 of the daily requirement for fiber.

Any type of bean is a superfood for diabetics. Your choices include black beans, navy, pinto or kidney beans. Beans are high in fiber and good source of potassium and magnesium. A half-cup serving of beans already gives 1/3 of the daily requirement for fiber.

Beans are classified as starchy vegetables but are also good protein sources. A half-cup serving can provide the same amount of proteins obtained from 1 ounce of meat. That without the saturated fats.

Beans do take some time to cook. Canned beans may be used to save time when cooking. Drain and rinse canned beans very well to remove most of the sodium.

GREEN LEAFY VEGETABLES

These are powerhouse foods rich in nutrients and antioxidants. These are also low in calories and in carbohydrate. That means that leafy greens can fill you up but will not raise your blood sugar levels too much.

CITRUS FRUITS

Citrus fruits like lime, lemon, grapefruit and oranges can do your blood sugar levels some good. These are high in soluble fiber that helps your body regulate the amount of sugar that gets absorbed in the blood. These sort of slow down how much sugar enters the blood, which helps to maintain the levels within normal range. Aside from fiber, you also get a good dose of vitamin C that strengthens the tissues against damage. Healthy tissues mean normal functioning and better regulatory mechanisms.

BERRIES

Berries are packed with antioxidants, along with an abundant supply of fiber and vitamins. You can eat them raw or cooked, included in various dishes such as whole grain breads. You can snack on a handful berries or add low fat yogurt and turn into a fruit salad or parfait. Smoothies are also a great way to get more berries. You can top berries on salads or cook and add as a dressing over meat dishes. There is an endless list of how you can add more berries in your diet.

TOMATOES

You get lots of vitamins E and C in tomatoes, along with iron and antioxidants. You get a great dose of lycopene, especially when you eat cooked tomatoes. This is a powerful antioxidant that can protect cells against damage. It can also help protect against cancers.

OMEGA-3 FATTY ACIDS

Fatty fishes are excellent sources of healthy fats called omega-3 fatty acids. These can reduce inflammation in the body that contributes to diabetes. It can also help the cells be more responsive to insulin, reducing insulin resistance linked to diabetes.

There are so many fishes you can choose from to get your daily dose of omega-3s. Choices include wild caught salmon, trout, tuna, mackerel and herring, among many others. These fishes are also great options to get your goal of eating around 6 to 9 ounces of fish weekly.

WHOLE GRAINS

Whole grains are the best choices because the nutrients you are after are contained in the bran and the germ. Refined grains have the bran and the germ removed, along with the nutrients. So if you eat refined grains, you are getting only the carbohydrates and the calories, and none of the nutrients you need. And carbohydrates wreck havoc on blood sugar levels. The same happens when you eat foods made with refined grains or flour.

The nutrients you get from whole grains include fiber, chromium, folate, omega-3 fatty acids and magnesium.

Great whole grain options include oatmeal and pearled barley, which are rich in potassium and fiber.

NUTS AND SEEDS

Nuts are another good source of fats. Why emphasis on fats? First, fats can help fill you up. It isn't just carbohydrates that can give you the energy you need. Fats can do that too. Not just that, energy from fats lasts longer than what you get from carbohydrates.

Aside from good fats, nuts are also good sources of fiber and magnesium. Some nuts also have the healthy omega-3 fats. Examples include flaxseeds and walnuts.

CHOCOLATE

Chocolate is not just pure pleasure. It is healthy too. Flavonoids are high in chocolates. These are phytonutrients that help reduce insulin resistance. These also help in improving the cells' sensitivity to insulin, making it easier to regulate blood sugar levels. Flavonoids also help in regulating the levels of insulin and in lowering the values of fasting blood glucose. Aside from all these, flavonoids in chocolate also help to curb cravings.

Do take care when choosing chocolates because not all kinds are good for diabetics. Milk chocolates are best avoided. These contain more milk and sugar than cocoa. Milk chocolates also have more fat and less flavonoids. The best chocolates to eat are dark chocolates, with at least 70% cocoa contents. According to research, people who ate dark chocolate had less urge to eat sweet, salty and/or fatty foods compared to those who ate milk chocolate. In one 2008 study conducted by the University of Copenhagen even found that people who ate dark chocolate had less appetite for pizza later in the day. Now that is a great way to control appetite for unhealthy foods.

Research has also found that flavonoids in chocolate promote more health benefits. It reduces the risk for stroke and heart attack, by as much as 2%. Blood pressure levels are also reduced down to normal range. Do you need more convincing to add dark chocolate to your daily menu?

BROCCOLI

This is a superhero food for diabetics. It is rich in sulforaphane, a compound that stimulates a number of anti-inflammatory processes. These processes improve blood sugar control. These also protect the lining of blood vessels, which often get damaged from the diabetic condition. In fact, the leading cause of death among diabetics is heart disease. This is why it is important to protect the cardiovascular system.

Sulforaphane has other health benefits as well. It initiates the body's natural detoxification mechanism and stimulates the enzymes that deactivate and alters the cancer-causing chemicals into harmless forms. In this new form, the body can effectively and easily remove from the body.

BLUEBERRIES

These plump, juicy berries are a powerhouse when it comes to health benefits. It has both types of fiber, insoluble and soluble. Insoluble fiber helps in flushing out fats and toxins out of the system by binding with these and facilitates faster passage through the intestinal tract. Soluble fiber helps in improving blood sugar control by slowing down carbohydrate digestion, thus, slowing down the release of sugar into the blood.

In a study conducted by the USDA, people who drank 2 ½ cup of juice from wild blueberries every day for 12 weeks experienced lowered blood sugar levels. Depression lessened and memory capabilities were enhanced with daily intake of blueberry juice. The major compound responsible for these effects are anthocyanins. These are compounds that give blueberry its color. It is found in abundance in the skin. Anthocyanins are antioxidants. These are natural chemicals that directly affects fat cells, causing them to shrink. This chemical can also trigger the release of the hormone adiponectin. This hormone also helps in the control of glucose levels in the blood. Higher levels of adiponectin in the body helps to increase the cells' sensitivity to the hormone insulin and keep the levels of blood sugar low.

OATMEAL

The most well-known benefit of oatmeal is in protecting the cardiovascular system from diseases and in lowering cholesterol levels in the body. But oatmeal's power as a superfood goes beyond the cardiovascular system.

Oatmeal is also effective in reducing your risk for type 2 diabetes. The large amounts of magnesium in oatmeal aids in more efficient use glucose and proper insulin release.

Steel-cut oatmeal is also easy to cook, much like quick-cooking oatmeal. This steel-cut version is more recommended because the grains are left whole. The nutrients, bound antioxidants and fiber are left intact, which allows you to get optimum benefits from each serving of oatmeal. The intact nutrients also make digestion a bit slower, which further regulates the amount of sugar (from digestion) that gets absorbed into the blood. This contributes to a more stable blood sugar level.

FISH

Fresh, wild caught fatty fishes contains a special kind of healthy fat that helps reduce the severity of diabetes symptoms and complications. This fat is omega-3 fatty acids. It reduces the inflammation in the body, which is a huge contributor to insulin resistance and diabetes. Thousands of research found that people with higher levels of omega-3 in the blood have lower systemic inflammation compared to those with lower omega-3 intake.

Eating a diet rich in fishes with omega-3 fats also have lower incidence of stroke. This condition is a common occurrence among diabetics. Stroke is a result of the negative impact of diabetes on the cardiovascular system. Eat fish that has been steamed, broiled or baked. Fried fish will increase your risk.

OLIVE OIL

In a recent Spanish study, those who included olive oil in their daily diet had 50% less chance of developing type 2 diabetes. This is a better outcome compared to when following low fat diet. In a study conducted by the University of Vienna and another one at the TUM (Technical University of Munich), olive oil improves the satiety from a meal compared to when using other oils like lard, canola (rapeseed) oil or butter.

Olive oil is a remarkable source of healthy monounsaturated fats. It is also rich in antioxidants. These natural compounds have protective functions on the cells, keeping them from oxidative damage. This effect protects against cardiovascular problems. This also helps reduce damage that promote inflammation, which in turn promotes insulin resistance and diabetes.

YOGURT

Yogurt, particularly Greek yogurt is good at better control over blood sugar levels. It has live probiotics that help improve the digestive functions. Most often, too much sugar in the body causes the microbiotics in the digestive tract to become unbalanced. This will further aid in insulin resistance and promote other processes that contribute to diabetes. By adding good probiotics through yogurt, balance is restored in the gut's microbiotic community.

Also, yogurt is a good source of healthy proteins. These proteins help in slowing down sugar conversion and absorption. This further helps in keeping the sugar levels in the blood more stable.

SPINACH

Leafy greens are excellent at reducing diabetes risk. One British study found that 1 serving of spinach every day had a 14% drop in diabetes risk. Spinach is rich in vitamin K and minerals such as folate, zinc, potassium, phosphorus and magnesium. An abundant supply of antioxidants such as different kinds of flavonoids and phytochemicals like zeaxanthin and lutein. Calcium is also abundant in spinach, so is the compound oxalic acid. This acid blocks the absorption of calcium from the leaves. To reduce the action of oxalic acid, blanch the spinach.

WALNUTS

This is one of the most widely cultivated tree nut worldwide. Walnuts are rich in alpha-linolenic acid, which is a kind of polyunsaturated fatty acid. This fatty acid can lower the degree of inflammation in the body. Again, inflammation plays a major role in diabetes. It contributes to insulin resistance and high levels of glucose in the blood.

Other compounds found in walnuts include omega-3 fatty acids, vitamin E, L-arginine and fiber. There is also an abundance of other important phytochemicals. All these play together to form a potent collection of natural chemicals to fight diabetes. These natural chemicals have antiviral, anti-cholesterol, anticancer and antioxidant.

These chemicals also halt the progression of diabetes and other chronic ailments.

QUINOA

This is actually more related to the leafy green spinach rather than grains but it looks and tastes like grain. Quinoa is packed with all the 9 essential amino acids. In a ½ cup serving of quinoa, 14 grams of proteins can be obtained.

One notable amino acid in quinoa is lysine. It enhances the absorption and action of calcium, particularly fat burning. It also works with carnitine, another nutrient that converts fatty acids into energy. Both of these functions contribute to reducing cholesterol in the body.

Quinoa is also packed with fiber. Per ½ cup serving of quinoa contains 2.6 grams of fiber. And by now, you already realize that fiber is integral to slowing down the entry of glucose into the blood to avoid rapid highs and lows that contribute to diabetes.

COLLARD GREENS

These are excellent natural sources of vitamin, another potent antioxidant in the body. Vitamin C aids in reducing the levels of cortisol in the body. It also aids in reducing inflammation as well.

Collard greens also have an abundant supply of ALA or alpha-lipoic acid. This is a micronutrient that has a profound effect in the body. It helps the body effectively deal with stress. There is another amazing action of ALA in the body. It stimulates the body to create its own supply of antioxidants. This effect was observed in a study by the Linus Pauling Institute scientists at Oregon State University. The creation of antioxidants by the body gives it a better chance at fighting damage from toxins and free radicals. The body is also helping itself to battle inflammation.

Aside from that, ALA can contribute to the reduction of blood sugar levels down to normal ranges. It also has supportive functions on the nerves, strengthening them from damage that leads to diabetic neuropathy.

Be careful when cooking collard greens. When overcooked, a strong sulfur smell is produced. Steam for only 5 minutes to keep the nutrients intact.

Bad Foods To Avoid If You Have Diabetes

Diabetics should avoid these foods because these can wreak havoc to blood sugar levels.

White Flour and White Rice

These contain large amounts of carbohydrates that are rapidly broken down and converted into sugar. These simple carbohydrates have high GI (glycemic index), which means these can cause your blood sugars to skyrocket in only a few minutes after eating. Avoid these at all cost.

White flour can be found in most baked breads and products, unless specifically stated that it used whole grains or whole wheat. All packaged baked goods also have white flour.

White Sugar

This is probably the most toxic food anyone can ever eat. It is high in calories, ultra high GI and nutritionally empty. It does nothing good in your body. This, along with white flour and white rice, is a major cause for insulin resistance and diabetes type 2.

Packaged Foods

These are unhealthy foods, whether you are diabetic or

not. It has loads of artificial ingredients that interfere with the normal and efficient regulatory mechanisms in the body. Some of these artificial compounds also interfere with cellular communication, which contributes to insulin resistance and poor blood glucose control.

Sugary Foods

Not all sweet foods are bad for diabetics. There are a handful of healthy ones, such as those from citrus fruits, a small serving of honey and berries.

Sugary foods that must be eliminated from the diet include all those made with white sugar and white flour. Examples are doughnuts, cakes, processed sugary snacks.

Fruit Juices

You should also avoid fruit juices. These may be freshly squeezed but in large amounts, the sugars can still affect the blood sugar levels. One reason is that fruit juices are stripped off of fiber. And without fiber, the natural fruit sugars are rapidly absorbed in the blood, causing spikes in both blood sugar and insulin levels. Commercial fruit juices and boxed juices are even more dangerous than freshly squeezed fruit juices. These contain tons of white sugar that wreak even more serious negative impact on blood sugar. And not to mention all the artificial ingredients added to make them stay fresh long while on the shelves.

Fried Foods

Foods cooked in tons of fats are always unhealthy. Also, deep frying heats up the oils for a long time. This will cause chemical changes in the structure of the oils, producing potentially dangerous toxins and compounds. These can trigger more inflammation, which will further worsen diabetes.

Also, too much oil in fried foods mean more calories. And more calories mean higher blood sugar levels.

And not to mention the trans fats. Most fast-food fried foods are cooked in trans fats. This is the unhealthiest fat in the world. It is highly altered and no longer contains any nutrients. Anything artificial worsens inflammation and diabetes as well.

Breakfast Recipes

Feta, Spinach and Tomato Strata

Superfoods: Tomatoes, Spinach

Servings: 6

Carbohydrates per serving: 27 g

Ingredients:

- 4 cups cubed whole-grain bread

- Nonstick cooking spray

- 1 pound fresh asparagus leaves, trimmed then sliced into 1-inch bits

- 2 cups fresh baby spinach

- 1 cup chopped onion

- 1 cup milk, fat-free

- 6 eggs

- 1/8 teaspoon black pepper, freshly ground

- 1/8 teaspoon salt

- 2 plum tomatoes, sliced thinly

- ¼ cup finely chopped fresh basil

- ½ cup feta cheese, reduced-fat

Directions:

- Spray a light coat of cooking oil on a rectangle baking dish.

- Place 2 cups of bread cubes on the baking and arrange in a single layer.

- Place onion and asparagus in a medium-sized saucepan. Add a small amount of boiling water and cook for 2-3 minutes until tender.

- Add spinach, give a quick stir and immediately drain.

- Place half of this spinach mixture over the bread cubes in the baking pan.

- Sprinkle the remaining bread cubes over and then the remaining spinach mixture.

- Get a large bowl and whisk milk and eggs together. Season with some pepper and salt.

- Pour the egg mixture over the bread and spinach in the baking dish.

- Get a spoon and use the back to lightly press down on the layers.

- Arrange the slices of tomatoes on top of the layers. Sprinkle feta and basil.

- Cover the baking dish with foil and chill in the fridge for 4-24 hours.

- Heat the oven up, 325 degrees.

- Bake the strata for 30 minutes with the foil still on.

- After 30 minutes, remove the foil and continue to bake for 40 minutes until the center of the dish reaches 180 degrees Fahrenheit. Expect that some liquid will still be present in the center. This will be fully absorbed as the dish sits.

- Let the dish stand for 10minutes before slicing and serving.

Nutritional Information:

- 247 calories

- 18 g proteins

- 419 mg sodium

- 9 g total fat, 3 g from saturated fat and 216 mg cholesterol

- 27 g carbohydrates, with 7 g from sugars and 7 g from fiber

Diabetic Exchanges:

- Vegetables: 1

- Starch: 1.5

- Medium Fat Meat: 1.5

Main Recipes

Salmon with Vegetable Bake

Superfoods: Salmon, Carrots, Olive Oil, Orange

Servings: 4

Carbohydrates per serving: 18 g

Ingredients:

- 1 pound skinless salmon fillets, 3/4 inch thickness

- 2 cups fresh mushrooms, sliced

- 2 cups thinly sliced carrot

- ½ cup sliced green onion

- 2 teaspoons snipped fresh oregano

- 2 teaspoons finely grated orange peel

- ¼ teaspoon salt

- 4 cloves garlic, sliced in half

- ¼ teaspoon whole black pepper

- 4 teaspoons olive oil

- 2 medium oranges, sliced thinly

- Salt and black pepper

- 4 sprigs fresh oregano

Directions:

- Cook carrots in a small amount of boiling water, in a covered saucepan until tender. Drain and transfer in a mixing bowl.

- Toss in green onions, oregano, mushrooms and orange peel. Add garlic and season with ¼ teaspoon of pepper and salt. Gently toss.

- Drizzle 1 teaspoon olive oil on each of the salmon fillet. Season with some pepper and salt, on each side of the fish.

- Create small foil packets by cutting heavy foil into 18 inches by 12 inches pieces.

- Place one fillet on a foil packet. Spoon some of the carrot mixture. Top with some orange slices and a sprig of oregano.

- Close the packets and fold the edges tightly to create a seal.

- Arrange the foil packets in a baking pan, in a single layer.

- Bake in a 350 degree preheated oven, until the fish flesh flakes easily with a fork and the carrots are tender.

- Open the packets to let some steam out. Transfer the fish and vegetables on separate serving plates and serve.

Nutritional Information:

- 252 calories

- 393 mg sodium

- 26 g proteins

- 10 g total fat, with 1 g from saturated fat

- 18 g carbohydrates, 12 g from sugars and 4 grams from fiber

Diabetic Exchanges:

- Lean meat: 3

- Fruit: 0.5

- Vegetables: 2

Quinoa with Avocado and Black Beans

Superfood: Beans, Quinoa

Servings: 6

Serving size: about 1 cup

Carbohydrates per serving: 39 grams

<u>Ingredients:</u>

- ¾ cup dried black beans

- 5 cups water

- 1 cup chopped onion

- Nonstick cooking spray

- 1 cup halved grape tomatoes

- ½ cup coarsely chopped fresh cilantro

- 1 teaspoon ground cumin

- 2 tablespoons fresh lime juice

- ½ teaspoon salt

- 1 tablespoon olive oil

- 2 cups cooked quinoa

- ¼ cup finely chopped fresh cilantro

- 1 tablespoon olive oil

- ¼ teaspoon salt

- 3 cups fresh spinach

- 1 medium-sized ripe avocado, peel and seed removed, meat sliced

- 1 medium lime, sliced into 6 wedges

Directions:

- Wash the beans and drain. Place in a large saucepan and pour 3 cups of water. Bring to a boil over medium high then lower heat to a simmer.

- Cook uncovered for 10 minutes. Remove the saucepan from heat and cover. Let it stand for about an hour before draining and rinsing.

- Spray a light coating of cooking spray on a slow cooker. Put the beans in.

- Add the remaining 2 cups of water.

- Add half of the tomatoes and onions. Sprinkle the cumin.

- Cover the slow cooker and cook set on low heat for 10 hours or on high heat for 5 hours until the beans turn soft. Turn off the heat.

- Add tomatoes, lime juice and ½ cup of cilantro. Season with pepper and salt. Drizzle 1 tablespoon of oil.

- Let the beans stand for a while to allow the flavors to mix and develop, at least 15 minutes.

- Toss quinoa and ¼ cup of cilantro. Season with salt and drizzle with a tablespoon of oil. Toss to mix well.

- Divide the spinach leaves into six and arrange a bed on each serving plate.

- Divide the quinoa mixture into 6 and arrange on top of the spinach leaves.

- Divide the bean mixture into 6 and carefully spoon a portion over the quinoa.

- Serve topped with avocado slices and a lime wedge.

Nutritional Information (per serving):

- 277 calories

- 11 g proteins

- 10 g total fat, 1 gram from saturated fat

- 39 g carbohydrates, 3 g from sugars and 9 grams from fiber

- 321 mg sodium

Diabetic Exchange:

- Vegetables: 1

- Starch: 2

- Lean Meat: 1

- Fat: 1

Snacks Recipes

Hot Trail Mix Cereal

Superfood: Nuts, Cereals, Flaxseed

Servings: 1

Carbohydrates per serving: 28 grams

Ingredients:

- ½ cup hot cooked cereal (such as hot wheat cereal)

- 2 tablespoons dry roasted mixed nuts

- 2 tablespoons mixed dried fruit bits

- 2 teaspoons flaxseed

Directions:

- Put the cereal in a serving bowl.

- Add the flaxseed, nuts and fruit bits on top. Serve and enjoy.

Nutritional Information:

- 227 calories

- 6 g proteins

- 28 g carbohydrates, 1 g from sugars and 4 g of fiber

- 16 mg sodium

- 11 g total fat, 1 g from saturated fat

Diabetic Exchanges:

- Fruit: 1

- Fat: 2

- Starch: 1

Dessert Recipes

Figs with Honey and Yogurt

Superfood: Yogurt

Servings: 2

Serving Size: 2/3 cup

Carbohydrates per serving: 24 grams

Ingredients:

- 1 8-oz carton low-fat plain yogurt

- 2 fresh figs, cut up

- ½ teaspoon vanilla

- 2 teaspoons honey

- 1 tablespoon toasted walnuts, coarsely chopped

Directions:

- Place a 100% cotton cheesecloth over a strainer. You may also use a coffee filter placed over a large mug. Pour the yogurt on the strainer (or coffee filter setup) and cover. Place in the refrigerator for 8-24 hours. The yogurt will form into a soft cheese as excess water drips through the cheesecloth/coffee filter.

- When ready, remove the thickened yogurt from the refrigerator. Discard the strained liquid.

- Place the yogurt in a mixing bowl. Stir in vanilla. Mix in the figs.

- Spoon the mixture into 2 dessert bowls. Sprinkle the walnuts in and drizzle with honey.

Nutritional Information (per serving):

- 157 calories

- 80 mg sodium

- 7 mg cholesterol

- 4 g total fat, 1 g from saturated fat

- 7 g protein

- 24 g carbohydrates, 2 grams from fiber

Diabetic Exchanges:

- Fruit: 1

- Fat: 1

- Milk: 0.5

Soup Recipes

Edamame and Vegetable Soup

Superfood: Edamame, Spinach, Broccoli

Servings: 8

Serving Size: ¾ cup

Carbohydrates per serving: 8 grams

<u>Ingredients</u>:

- ½ cup chopped onion

- 1 tablespoon canola oil

- 4 garlic cloves, minced

- 2 cups chicken broth (reduced-sodium kind)

- 1 cup edamame (sweet soybeans), shelled

- 1 ½ cups small broccoli florets

- 1 12.3–oz. package firm light tofu, silken-style

- 1 9-oz. package fresh spinach leaves

- 1 6-oz. container plain Greek yogurt, fat-free

- ½ teaspoon fresh ground black pepper

- ½ teaspoon salt

- 2 tablespoons snipped fresh chives

- ¼ cup roasted soy nuts, unsalted

Directions:

- Sauté garlic and onions in oil, in a large Dutch oven, until tender. Remove garlic and onions and set aside.

- Pour the broth into the same Dutch oven and bring to a boil over medium high heat.

- Add edamame and broccoli florets. When the soup boils again, reduce heat to a simmer. Cook uncovered until the florets are tender. Remove and transfer the edamame and broccoli to a large mixing bowl and set them aside. Use a slotted spoon for this.

- Add the spinach leaves into the broth in the Dutch oven. Cook until the leaves start to wilt.

- Remove the Dutch oven from the heat and slightly cool.

- Stir in the onion mixture and broccoli mixture.

- Add tofu and half of the spinach soup in a food

processor and pulse until smooth. Pour back into the Dutch oven.

- Add yogurt. Season with pepper and salt.

- Cover and cook on medium low until just heated through. Stir occasionally.

- Ladle the soup into servings bowls. Serve topped with chives and toasted soy nuts.

Nutritional Information (per serving):

- 106 calories

- 362 mg sodium

- 11 g proteins

- 8 g carbohydrates: 3 g sugar, 3 g fiber

- 4 g total fat

Diabetic exchange:

- Starch: 0.5

- Consider as free exchange: 0

- Lean meat: 1.5

Salad Recipes

Superfoods Salad

Superfoods: Spinach, Blueberries, Strawberries, Raspberries, Walnuts

Servings: 4

Serving size: 2 cups

Carbohydrates per serving: 22 grams

<u>Ingredients:</u>

- 1/3 cup raspberry vinegar
- 2 tablespoons honey
- 2 tablespoons minced fresh mint
- ¼ teaspoon salt
- 1 tablespoon canola oil
- 2 cups chicken breast, cooked and chopped
- 4 cups fresh baby spinach leaves
- ½ cup fresh blueberries
- 2 cups fresh strawberries, hulls removed, sliced

- ¼ cup toasted walnuts, coarsely chopped

- ½ teaspoon fresh ground black pepper

- 1 ounce crumbled semi-soft goat cheese

Directions:

- Make the vinaigrette by placing vinegar, honey, salt, oil and mint in a screw-lid jar. Close tightly and shake well. Or, you simply whisk all the vinaigrette ingredients in a bowl. Set aside.

- Get a large mixing bowl and place chicken, goat cheese, walnuts, spinach, blueberries and strawberries. Toss to mix everything.

- Divide the salad into 4 and spoon each portion on serving plates. Drizzle a few teaspoons of the prepared vinaigrette. Sprinkle with freshly ground pepper.

Nutritional Information:

- 303 calories

- 26 g protein

- 249 g sodium

- 63 mg cholesterol

- 13 g total fat, with 2 g from saturated fat

- 22 g carbohydrates, with 14 g from sugars and 3 g from fiber

Diabetic Exchanges:

- Fruit: 0.5

- Other carbohydrates: 0.5

- Lean Meat: 3.5

- Fat: 2

- Vegetables: 1

Drinks Recipes

Carrot Smoothie

Superfoods: Carrots, Oranges

Servings: 3

Serving size: 5 ounces

Carbohydrates per serving: 13 g

Ingredients:

- 1 cup carrots, sliced

- ½ teaspoon orange peel, finely shredded

- 1 ½ cups ice cubes

- 1 cup orange juice

- Orange peel curls (optional)

Directions:

- Place carrots and a small amount of boiling water in a small saucepan. Cover and cook until the carrots become very tender. Drain and set aside to cool.

- Once cooled, place carrots in a blender or food

processor. Add orange juice and orange peel.

- Blend until everything is smooth.

- Put the ice cubes in the blender or food processor. Pulse until smooth.

- Get serving glasses and pour the carrot smoothie.

Nutritional Information:

- 55 calories

- 1 g protein

- 13 g carbohydrates, 1 g from fiber

- 16 mg sodium

Diabetic Exchange:

- Fruit: 0.5

- Vegetables: 0.5

Conclusion

Thank you again for reading this book!

I hope this book was able to help you to understand what you need to do to reverse the effects of diabetes.

The next step is to make sure that you follow what's written in this book so you can effectively fight diabetes and live a stress-free, happy life!

Finally, if you enjoyed this book, then I'd like to ask you for a favor, would you be kind enough to leave a review for this book on Amazon? It'd be greatly appreciated!

Thank you and good luck!

Check Out My Other Books

Below you'll find some of my other popular books that are popular on Amazon and Kindle as well.

<u>Autism: Simple And Inexpensive Autism Therapies</u>

You can simply search for these titles on the Amazon website to find them.

www.ingramcontent.com/pod-product-compliance
Lightning Source LLC
Chambersburg PA
CBHW071230280526
45787CB00002B/872